The meal will taste much more [divine]
With some tomatoes from the [vine.]
I pick them fresh; they taste so fine!
A salsa fresca will be mine.

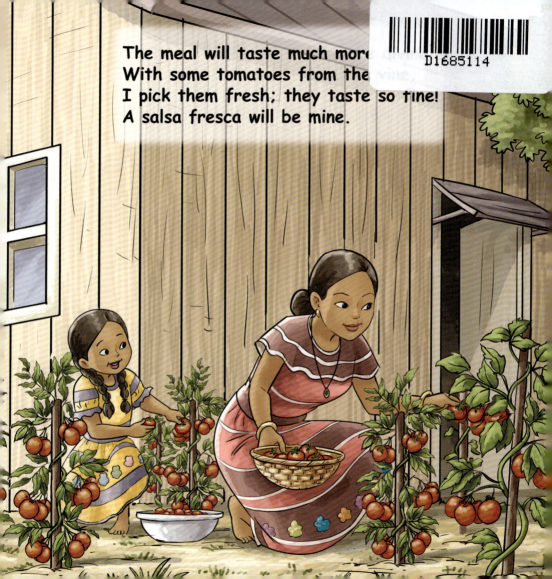

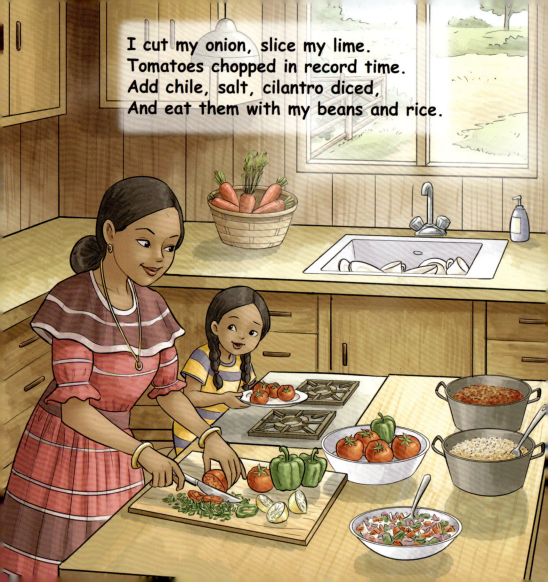

I cut my onion, slice my lime.
Tomatoes chopped in record time.
Add chile, salt, cilantro diced,
And eat them with my beans and rice.

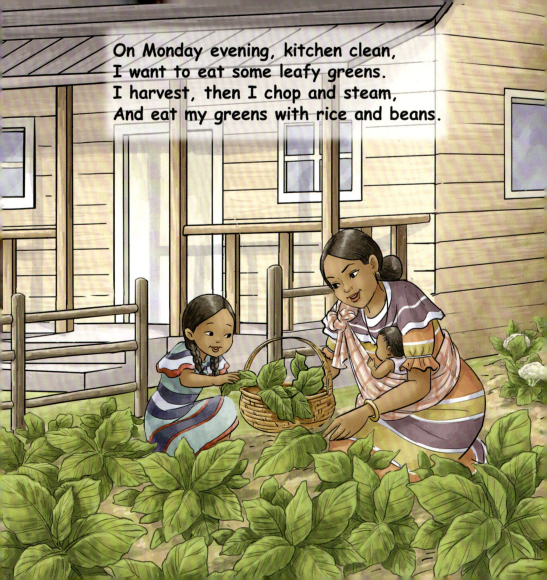

On Monday evening, kitchen clean,
I want to eat some leafy greens.
I harvest, then I chop and steam,
And eat my greens with rice and beans.

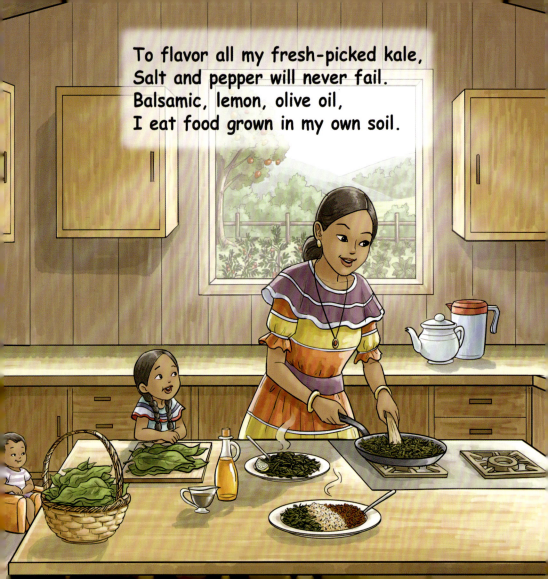

To flavor all my fresh-picked kale,
Salt and pepper will never fail.
Balsamic, lemon, olive oil,
I eat food grown in my own soil.

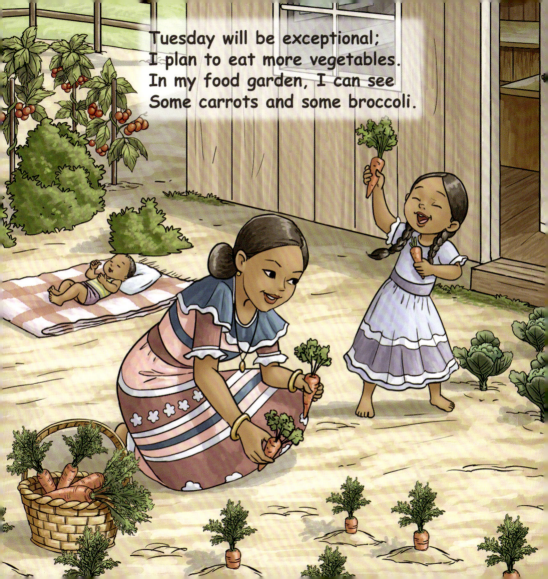

Tuesday will be exceptional;
I plan to eat more vegetables.
In my food garden, I can see
Some carrots and some broccoli.

When my veggies are chopped and sliced,
I cook them with my beans and rice.
Then, I'll add some avocado;
Save some for my lunch tomorrow.

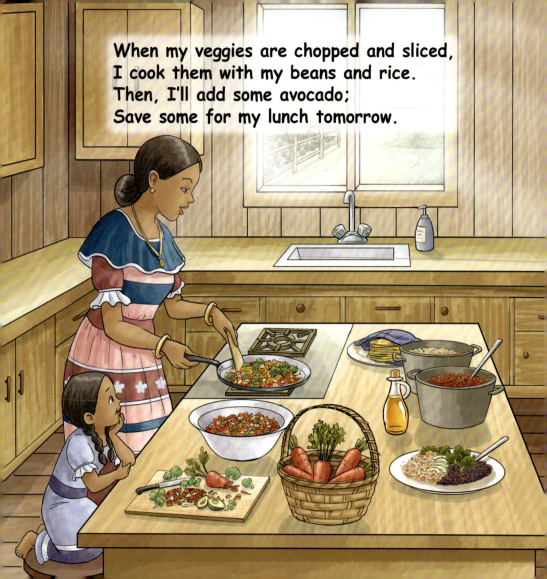

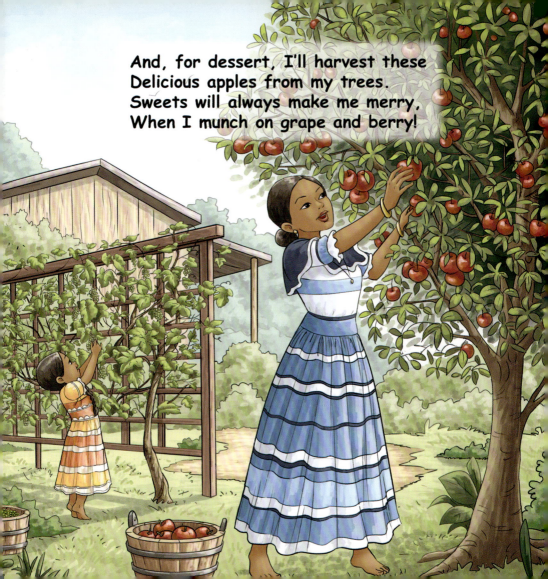

And, for dessert, I'll harvest these
Delicious apples from my trees.
Sweets will always make me merry,
When I munch on grape and berry!

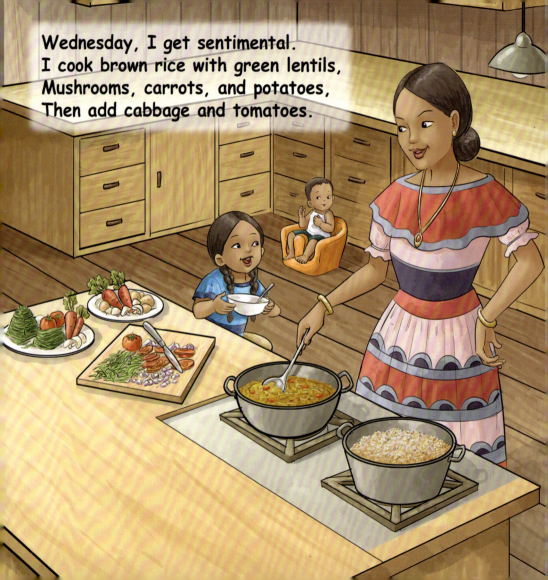

Wednesday, I get sentimental.
I cook brown rice with green lentils,
Mushrooms, carrots, and potatoes,
Then add cabbage and tomatoes.

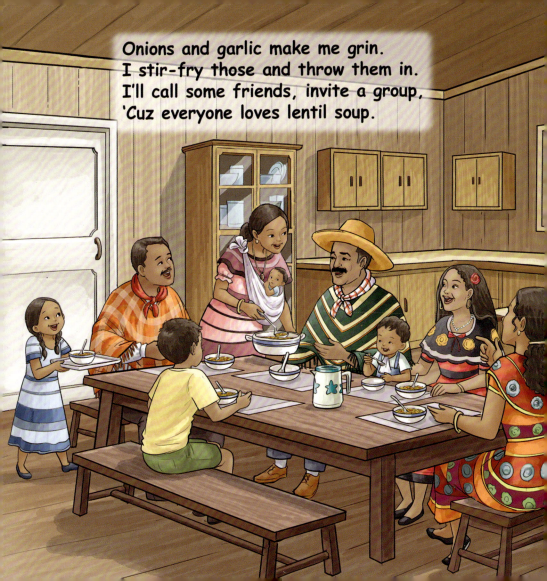

Onions and garlic make me grin.
I stir-fry those and throw them in.
I'll call some friends, invite a group,
'Cuz everyone loves lentil soup.

On Thursday, I can use a rest,
So warmed leftovers work the best.
Reheat the lentils and the rice;
Sprinkle with cheese. It tastes so nice!

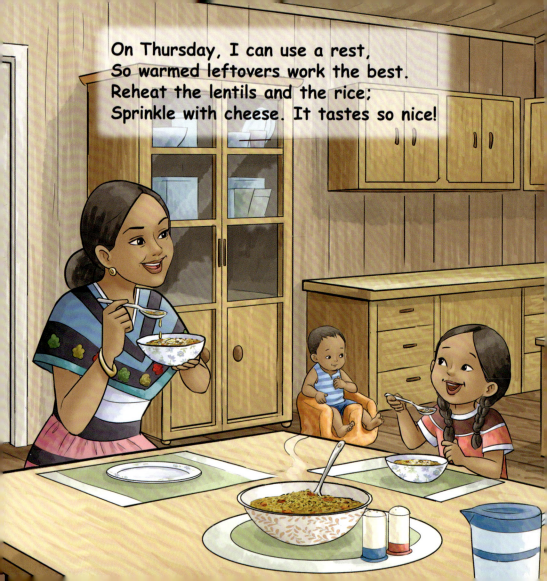

On Friday, I've got bigger plans,
With cauliflower baked in pans.
Winter squash and black beans added;
And a tasty garden salad.

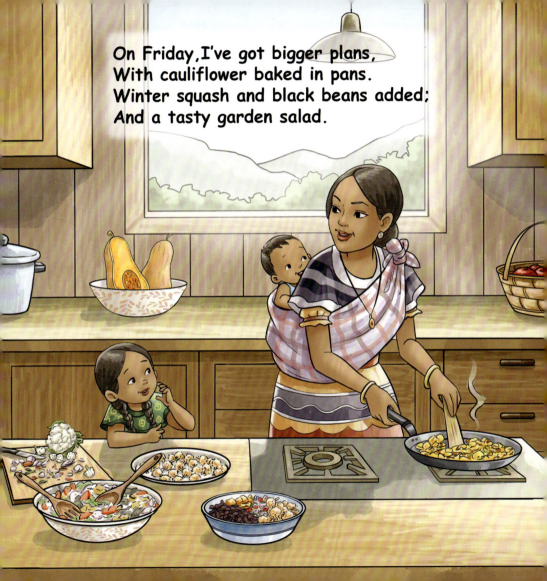

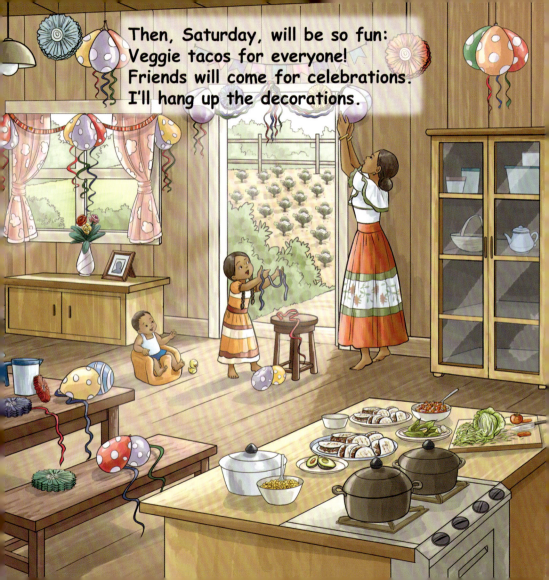

Then, Saturday, will be so fun:
Veggie tacos for everyone!
Friends will come for celebrations.
I'll hang up the decorations.

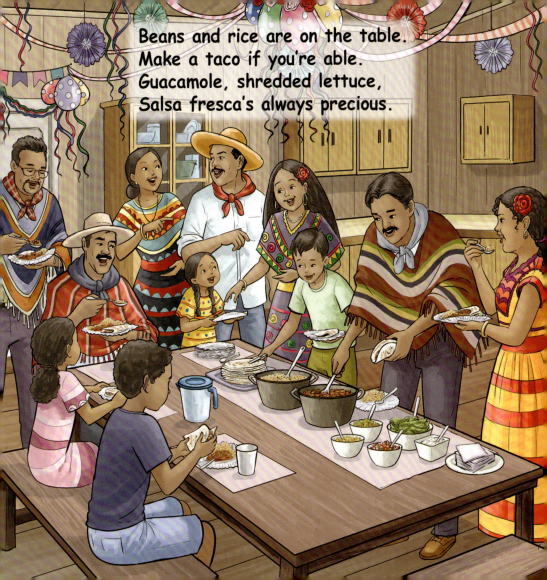

Beans and rice are on the table.
Make a taco if you're able.
Guacamole, shredded lettuce,
Salsa fresca's always precious.

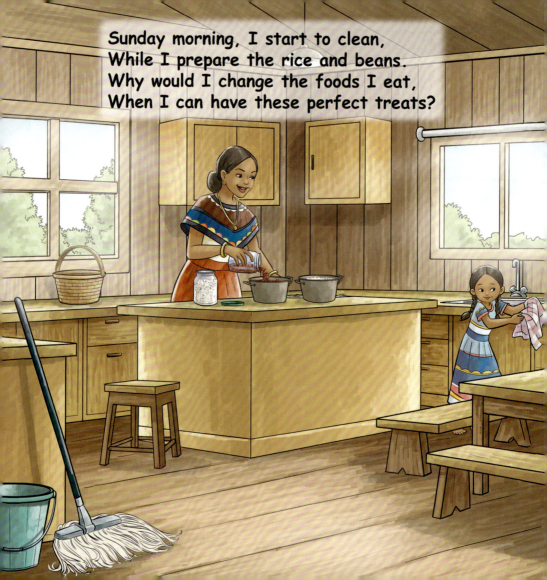

Sunday morning, I start to clean,
While I prepare the rice and beans.
Why would I change the foods I eat,
When I can have these perfect treats?

I keep my food healthy and cheap,
I cook in bulk to start the week.
Let's love the earth and treat it right.
Please keep on eating beans and rice!

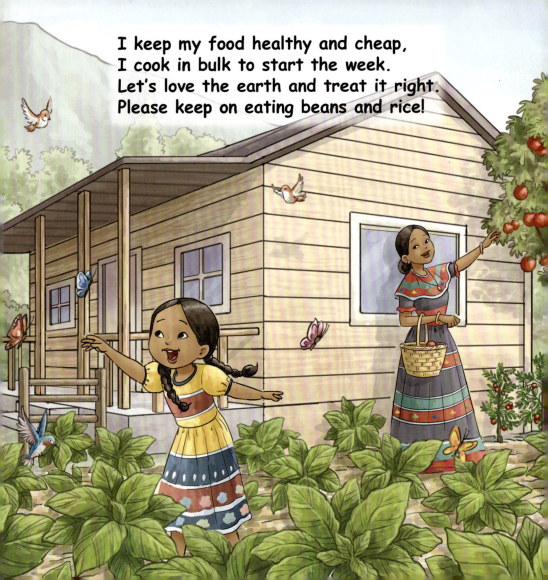

Other books by this author

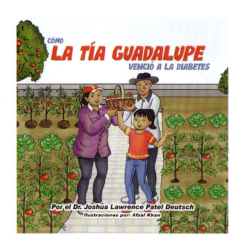

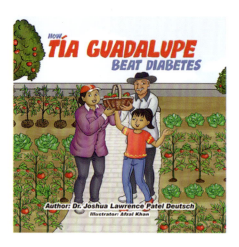

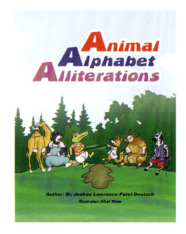

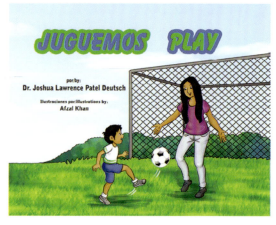